# THE COMPLETE PCOS DIET COOKBOOK FOR BEGINNERS

Nourish Your Way To well-being With The Ultimate Recipes Crafted To Soothe Symptoms, Balance Hormones, and Enhance Fertility

**BY**

**Mildred Kent**

# Copyright Notice

# TABLE OF CONTENT

# INTRODUCTION

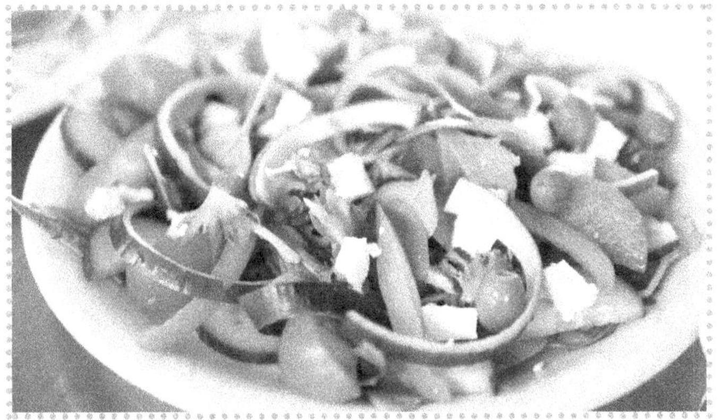

Introduction to PCOS Diet Cookbook for Beginners

The Ultimate "PCOS Diet Cookbook for Beginners"! If you've been diagnosed with Polycystic Ovary Syndrome (PCOS), you're not alone. Many women face this condition and the unique challenges it presents. This book aims to help you navigate these challenges by providing you with the tools and knowledge needed to manage PCOS through diet.

Eating the right foods can have a significant impact on managing PCOS symptoms and improving your overall health. This cookbook is designed to make the transition to a PCOS-friendly diet as easy and delicious as possible. From understanding what PCOS is to discovering the best foods to eat, this book will guide you step by step.

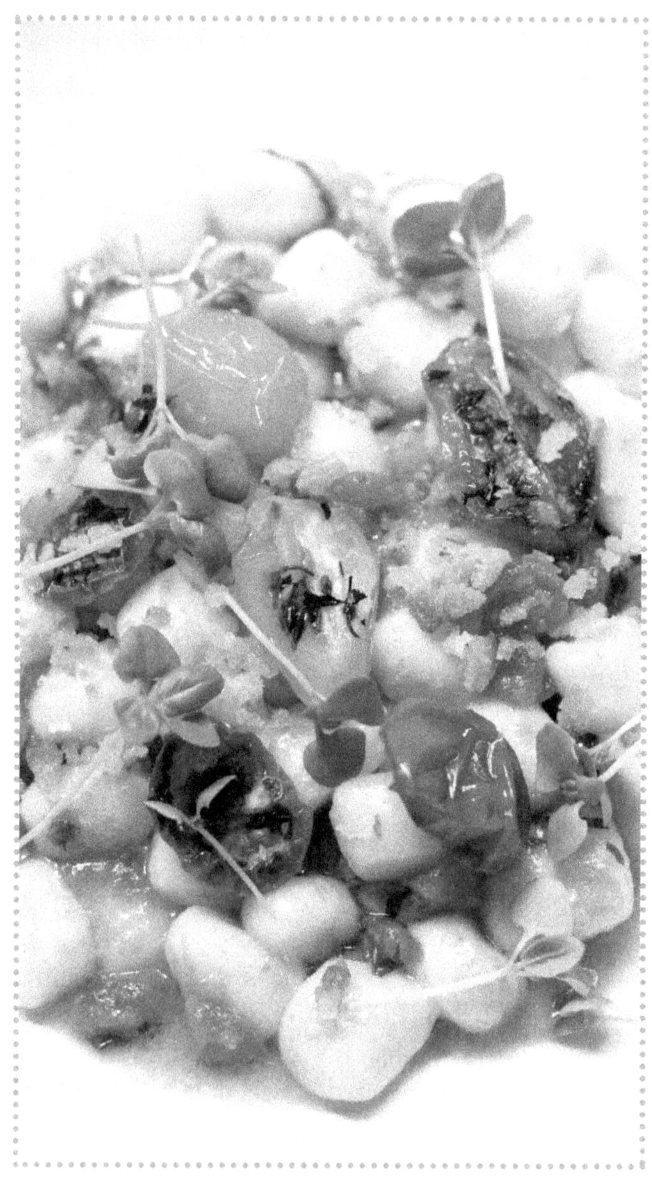

# CHAPTER ONE

## Understanding PCOS

### 1.1   What is PCOS?

PCOS is a hormonal condition that is commonly experienced by women who are fertile. Polycystic ovaries, high androgen levels, and irregular menstrual periods are its defining features. Understanding the basics of PCOS is crucial for managing it effectively.

PCOS can lead to various health issues, including infertility, insulin resistance, and an increased risk of diabetes. While the exact cause of PCOS is unknown, genetics and lifestyle factors play a significant role.

## 1.2 Symptoms and Diagnosis

PCOS symptoms can vary greatly, but frequently include:

1.  Irregular periods or no periods at all

2.  Excess hair growth (hirsutism) on the face, chest, or back

3.  Acne and oily skin

4.  Weight gain, especially around the abdomen

5.  Thinning hair or hair loss on the scalp

6.  Difficulty getting pregnant

Diagnosing PCOS typically involves a combination of medical history, physical examination, blood tests to measure hormone levels, and an ultrasound to check for cysts on the ovaries.

## 1.3    The Role of Diet in Managing PCOS

Diet plays a vital role in managing PCOS symptoms. Since many women with PCOS have insulin resistance, it's important to focus on foods that help regulate blood sugar levels. A balanced diet can help manage weight, reduce symptoms, and improve overall health.

Foods rich in fiber, lean proteins, and healthy fats can help maintain stable blood sugar levels and improve insulin sensitivity. Avoiding processed foods, sugary snacks, and refined carbohydrates is equally important in managing PCOS.

## 1.4    Importance of a Balanced Diet

A balanced diet is essential for everyone, but it's especially crucial for those with PCOS. Eating a variety of nutrient-dense foods ensures you're getting the vitamins and minerals your body needs to function properly.

Incorporating a mix of fruits, vegetables, whole grains, lean proteins, and healthy fats into your diet can help alleviate PCOS symptoms and promote overall well-being. This book will provide you with practical tips and delicious recipes to help you achieve a balanced diet tailored to managing PCOS.

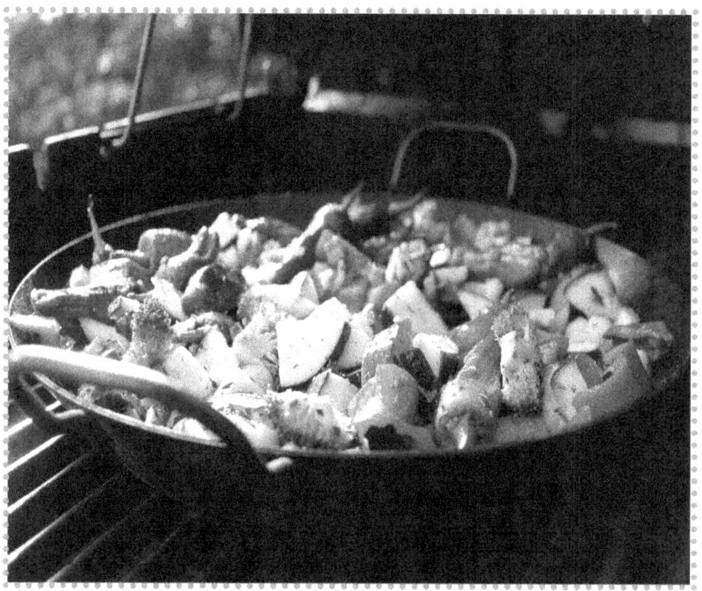

# CHAPTER TWO

## PCOS-Friendly Foods

Now that we understand the importance of diet in managing PCOS, let's dive into the specific foods that can help you on your journey to better health.

## 2.1 Nutrients Essential for Managing PCOS

Certain nutrients are particularly beneficial for managing PCOS:

1. ****Structure**:** promotes the health of the digestive system and aids in blood sugar regulation. Found in fruits, vegetables, whole grains, and legumes.

2. ****Omega-3 Fatty Acids**:** Reduce inflammation and improve insulin sensitivity. Found in fatty fish, flaxseeds, and walnuts.

3.  **Magnesium:** Helps with insulin sensitivity and reduces inflammation. Found in leafy greens, nuts, and seeds.

4.  **Vitamin D:** Supports hormonal balance and improves insulin resistance. Found in fatty fish, fortified foods, and sun exposure.

5.  **Antioxidants:** Combat oxidative stress and inflammation. Found in berries, leafy greens, nuts, and seeds.

## 2.2  Best Foods for PCOS: Fruits, Vegetables, and Whole Grains

Incorporating a variety of fruits, vegetables, and whole grains into your diet is crucial for managing PCOS:

1.  **Fruits:** Berries, apples, pears, and citrus fruits are high in fiber and antioxidants.

2.  **Vegetables:** Leafy greens, cruciferous vegetables, and colorful veggies provide essential vitamins and minerals.

3.  **Whole Grains**:** Brown rice, quinoa, oats, and whole wheat products offer fiber and nutrients without causing blood sugar spikes.

## 2.3. Protein Sources: Lean Meats, Fish, and Plant-Based Options

Protein keeps you feeling full and is essential for muscle growth and repair:

1.  **Lean Meats**:** High-quality protein without added fat can be found in chicken, turkey, and lean beef or pork chops.

2  **A fish**:** Salmon, mackerel, and sardines are among the fatty fish that are great providers of omega-3 fatty acids.

3.  **Plant-Based Proteins**:** Beans, lentils, tofu, and tempeh are great alternatives to animal proteins and are rich in fiber.

## 2.4 Healthy Fats: Oils, Nuts, and Seeds

Good fats are necessary for the synthesis of hormones and general health:

1.  **Oils:** Olive oil, avocado oil, and coconut oil are good sources of healthy fats.

2.  **Nuts:** Almonds, walnuts, and pistachios offer healthy fats, fiber, and protein.

3.  **Seeds:** Chia seeds, flaxseeds, and pumpkin seeds are rich in omega-3s and other essential nutrients.

By incorporating these PCOS-friendly foods into your diet, you can take control of your health and manage your symptoms more effectively. The recipes and tips in this book will make it easy and enjoyable to eat in a way that supports your well-being. Let's embark on this journey together!

# CHAPTER THREE

## Foods to Avoid

Managing PCOS effectively often involves making significant dietary changes. Certain foods can exacerbate symptoms and hinder progress, so it's essential to know what to avoid. This chapter focuses on key food groups and substances that can negatively impact PCOS.

## 3.1    Refined Carbohydrates and Sugars

Refined carbohydrates and sugars can cause rapid spikes in blood sugar levels, leading to increased insulin resistance, a common issue in women with PCOS. Foods high in refined carbs and sugars include:

1.   **White Bread and Pasta:** Made from refined flour, these foods lack fiber and essential nutrients, causing blood sugar levels to spike.

2. **Sugary Snacks and Desserts:** Cookies, cakes, candies, and pastries are loaded with sugars and unhealthy fats.

3. **Sweetened Beverages:** Sodas, fruit juices, and energy drinks often contain high amounts of added sugars.

Avoiding these foods can help stabilize blood sugar levels and improve insulin sensitivity, crucial for managing PCOS symptoms.

## 3.2    Processed Foods and Trans Fats

Processed foods often contain unhealthy additives, preservatives, and trans fats, which can contribute to inflammation and worsen PCOS symptoms. Common processed foods to avoid include:

1. **Fast Food:** Burgers, fries, and fried chicken are typically high in trans fats and sodium.

2. **Packaged Snacks:** Chips, crackers, and microwave popcorn often contain trans fats and artificial ingredients.

3.  **Frozen Meals**:** Many frozen dinners are high in sodium, preservatives, and unhealthy fats.

Trans fats, found in many processed foods, can increase inflammation and disrupt hormonal balance. Reading labels and choosing whole, unprocessed foods can help reduce intake of these harmful substances.

## 3.3   Dairy and Its Impact on PCOS

Dairy products can affect PCOS symptoms due to their potential impact on hormone levels. Some women with PCOS may be sensitive to dairy, leading to increased inflammation and insulin resistance. Dairy products to consider limiting include:

1.  **Whole Milk**:** High in saturated fat and can exacerbate insulin resistance.

2.  **Cheese**:** Often high in fat and calories.

3. **Ice Cream and Yogurt**: Many are loaded with added sugars.

While not all women with PCOS need to eliminate dairy completely, reducing intake or opting for dairy alternatives like almond milk or coconut yogurt can be beneficial.

## 3.4  Caffeine and Alcohol: Moderation Tips

Caffeine and alcohol can impact PCOS symptoms if consumed in excess. Moderation is key:

1. **Caffeine**: Found in coffee, tea, and certain sodas, excessive caffeine can disrupt sleep and increase stress, which may worsen PCOS symptoms. Limiting caffeine intake to one or two cups of coffee per day can help.

2. **Alcohol**: Alcohol can affect blood sugar levels and hormone balance. Drinking in moderation, such as one drink per day for women, is recommended. Opting for red wine over sugary cocktails is a better choice.

By avoiding or moderating these foods and substances, you can better manage PCOS symptoms and support your overall health.

# CHAPTER FOUR

## Setting Up Your PCOS Diet Kitchen

Creating a kitchen environment that supports your PCOS-friendly diet is crucial for long-term success. This chapter will guide you through essential kitchen tools, pantry staples, meal planning tips, and how to read nutrition labels for PCOS-friendly choices.

## 4.1 Essential Kitchen Tools and Equipment

Having the right tools and equipment can make meal preparation easier and more enjoyable. Essential items include:

1. **Sharp Knives and Cutting Boards:** For efficient chopping and slicing of fruits, vegetables, and proteins.

2.   **Blender or Food Processor:** Ideal for making smoothies, purees, and healthy sauces.

3.   **Non-Stick Cookware:** Reduces the need for added fats when cooking.

4.   **Measuring Cups and Spoons:** Ensures accurate portion sizes and ingredient measurements.

5.   **Storage Containers:** For meal prepping and storing leftovers.

These tools will help you prepare nutritious meals quickly and efficiently, making it easier to stick to your PCOS diet.

## 4.2    Stocking Your Pantry: Staples and Fresh Ingredients

Stocking your pantry with PCOS-friendly staples ensures you always have healthy options available. Key items include:

1. **Whole Grains:** Brown rice, quinoa, oats, and whole wheat products.

2. **Legumes:** Beans, lentils, and chickpeas for protein and fiber.

3. **Nuts and Seeds:** Almonds, walnuts, chia seeds, and flaxseeds for healthy fats and nutrients.

4. **Healthy Oils:** Olive oil, coconut oil, and avocado oil for cooking and dressings.

5. **Spices and Herbs:** Turmeric, cinnamon, basil, and rosemary for adding flavor without extra calories.

Fresh ingredients to keep on hand include a variety of fruits, vegetables, lean proteins (such as chicken and fish), and plant-based proteins like tofu and tempeh.

## 4.3    Meal Planning and Preparation Tips

Effective meal planning and preparation can help you stay on track with your PCOS diet. Tips include:

1.   **Make a Meal Plan:** Make a menu for breakfast, lunch, dinner, and snacks each week. Take into account your timetable and select dishes that work within your limits.

2.   **Prep in Advance:** Chop vegetables, cook grains, and prepare proteins in advance to save time during the week.

3.   **Batch Cooking:** Prepare large batches of soups, stews, and casseroles that can be portioned and frozen for later use.

4.   **Use Leftovers:** Repurpose leftovers into new meals to reduce waste and save time.

By planning and preparing your meals in advance, you can ensure you always have healthy options available, making it easier to stick to your diet.

## 4.4    Reading Nutrition Labels for PCOS-Friendly Choices

Comprehending nutrition labels is vital for creating knowledgeable food selections. Key points to look for include:

1. **Serving Size:** Check the serving size and compare it to the amount you plan to eat.

2. **Calories and Macronutrients:** Monitor calorie intake and ensure a balance of carbohydrates, proteins, and fats.

3. **Ingredients List:** Avoid products with added sugars, trans fats, and artificial ingredients.

4. **Fiber Content:** Choose foods high in fiber to help manage blood sugar levels.

By learning to read and understand nutrition labels, you can make healthier choices that support your PCOS management goals.

Setting up your kitchen for success, stocking it with PCOS-friendly foods, and planning your meals effectively can make a significant difference in managing PCOS. The following chapters will

provide you with delicious recipes and further tips
to help you on your journey.

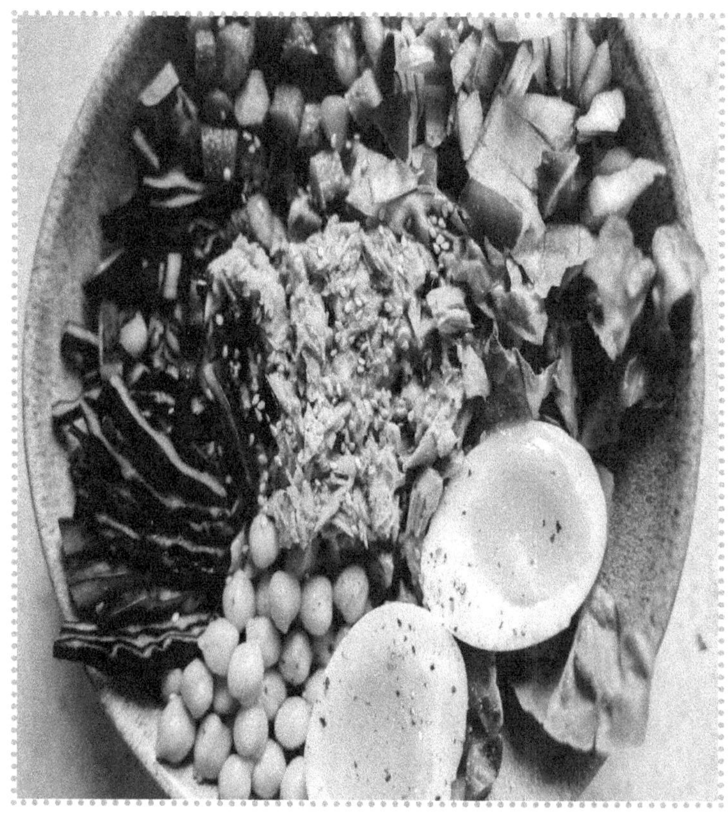

# CHAPTER FIVE

## Breakfast Recipes

There's a good reason why breakfast is frequently referred to as the most significant meal of the day. Starting your day with a nutritious, well-balanced breakfast can set the tone for the rest of your day, helping to stabilize blood sugar levels and keep energy levels high. For women with PCOS, this is especially important. This chapter will guide you through a variety of breakfast options that are quick, easy, and tailored to support your health.

## 5.1  Quick and Easy Morning Meals

Mornings can be hectic, but that doesn't mean you have to skip breakfast or settle for something unhealthy. Here are some quick and easy breakfast ideas that are perfect for busy mornings:

## 1. Avocado Toast with a Twist

Avocado toast is a popular breakfast choice that's both delicious and nutritious. For a PCOS-friendly twist, top your whole grain toast with mashed avocado, a sprinkle of chia seeds, and a drizzle of olive oil. Add a poached egg on top for an extra boost of protein.

## 2. Greek Yogurt Parfait

A Greek yogurt parfait is a quick and easy breakfast that can be made in minutes. Arrange Greek yogurt, fresh berries, granola, and honey drizzled over top. Probiotics included in Greek yogurt are abundant and good for your intestines.

## 3. Overnight Oats

Overnight oats are a great option for busy mornings because they can be prepared the night before. Combine rolled oats, almond milk, chia seeds, and a touch of maple syrup in a jar. Let it sit in the refrigerator overnight. Sprinkle some cinnamon, almonds, and fresh fruit on top in the morning.

## 4. Banana and Nut Butter Toast

Spread a layer of your favorite nut butter on a slice of whole grain toast and top with sliced bananas. Sprinkle with flaxseeds for added fiber and omega-3 fatty acids. This breakfast is quick, easy, and provides a good balance of protein, healthy fats, and carbohydrates.

## 5.2    Smoothies and Shakes

Smoothies and shakes are perfect for a quick, on-the-go breakfast. They are versatile and can be packed with nutrients to help manage PCOS symptoms. Here are some delicious and nutritious smoothie and shake recipes:

## 1. Green Power Smoothie

Blend together a handful of spinach, a frozen banana, a scoop of protein powder, a tablespoon of almond butter, and a cup of almond milk. This smoothie is packed with vitamins, minerals, and protein to keep you energized throughout the morning.

## 2. Berry Blast Smoothie

Combine frozen mixed berries, Greek yogurt, a tablespoon of chia seeds, and a cup of unsweetened coconut milk in a blender. Blend until smooth. This smoothie is high in antioxidants and fiber, which are beneficial for managing PCOS symptoms.

## 3. Chocolate Peanut Butter Protein Shake

For a more indulgent yet healthy option, blend together a scoop of chocolate protein powder, a tablespoon of peanut butter, a frozen banana, and a cup of unsweetened almond milk. This shake is rich in protein and healthy fats, making it a satisfying breakfast option.

## 4. Tropical Mango Smoothie

Blend together frozen mango chunks, a tablespoon of flaxseeds, a scoop of vanilla protein powder, and a cup of coconut water. This tropical smoothie is refreshing and provides a good source of fiber and omega-3 fatty acids.

## 5.3    High-Protein and Fiber-Rich Options

Protein and fiber are essential components of a PCOS-friendly diet. They prolong the sense of fullness and assist to normalize blood sugar levels. Here are some high-protein and fiber-rich breakfast ideas:

## 1. Scrambled Eggs with Veggies

Scrambled eggs are a classic high-protein breakfast. For a PCOS-friendly twist, add a variety of colorful vegetables like bell peppers, spinach, and tomatoes. For extra fiber, serve with a slice of whole grain toast.

## 2. Quinoa Breakfast Bowl

A multipurpose grain that is rich in fiber and protein is quinoa. Cook quinoa according to package instructions and top with sautéed vegetables, a poached egg, and a drizzle of tahini.

This savory breakfast bowl is both satisfying and nutritious.

## 3. Chia Seed Pudding

Omega-3 fatty acids and fiber abound in chia seeds. To make chia seed pudding, combine chia seeds with almond milk and a touch of vanilla extract. Let it sit in the refrigerator overnight. In the morning, top with fresh fruit and a sprinkle of nuts.

## 4. Cottage Cheese and Fruit

Cottage cheese is high in protein and pairs well with fresh fruit. For a quick and easy breakfast, top a bowl of cottage cheese with sliced strawberries, blueberries, and a drizzle of honey. For added crunch and good fats, add a handful of nuts.

## 5.4 Gluten-Free and Dairy-Free Breakfast Ideas

For those with dietary restrictions or sensitivities, here are some gluten-free and dairy-free breakfast options that are both delicious and PCOS-friendly:

## 1. Gluten-Free Pancakes

Make gluten-free pancakes using almond flour or a gluten-free pancake mix. Top with fresh fruit, a dollop of coconut yogurt, and a drizzle of pure maple syrup. These pancakes are light, fluffy, and free from gluten and dairy.

## 2. Smoothie Bowl

A smoothie bowl is a thicker version of a smoothie that's eaten with a spoon. Blend together frozen berries, a banana, and coconut milk until smooth. Transfer into a bowl, then garnish with sliced fruit, granola, and chia seeds.

## 3. Tofu Scramble

An excellent plant-based substitute for scrambled eggs is tofu scramble. Crumble firm tofu into a skillet and sauté with turmeric, garlic powder, and a variety of vegetables. Serve with gluten-free toast or a side of avocado.

## 4. Grain-Free Breakfast Muffins

Make a batch of grain-free breakfast muffins using almond flour, eggs, and shredded zucchini. These muffins are not only gluten-free and dairy-free, but they're also packed with nutrients. Enjoy them fresh out of the oven or as a quick grab-and-go breakfast.

# CHAPTER SIX

## Lunch Recipes

A nutritious lunch is important for maintaining energy levels and managing PCOS symptoms throughout the day. This chapter offers a variety of satisfying salads, hearty soups and stews, delicious sandwiches and wraps, and vegetarian and vegan options.

## 6.1 Satisfying Salads

Salads can be a great way to get a variety of nutrients in one meal. Here are some satisfying salad recipes that are perfect for lunch:

### 1. Mediterranean Chickpea Salad

Combine chickpeas, cherry tomatoes, cucumber, red onion, and kalamata olives in a bowl. Toss with a dressing made from olive oil, lemon juice, and oregano. Top with crumbled feta cheese for a Mediterranean twist.

## 2. Quinoa and Black Bean Salad

Mix cooked quinoa, black beans, corn, red bell pepper, and avocado in a large bowl. Add a dash of cumin, olive oil, and lime juice for dressing. This salad is high in protein and fiber, making it a satisfying lunch option.

## 3. Kale and Apple Salad

Toss chopped kale with thinly sliced apples, dried cranberries, and toasted almonds. Dress with a simple vinaigrette made from apple cider vinegar, olive oil, and honey. This salad is packed with vitamins and antioxidants.

## 4. Chicken Caesar Salad

For a protein-packed lunch, combine romaine lettuce, grilled chicken breast, and cherry tomatoes. Top with a homemade Caesar dressing made from Greek yogurt, lemon juice, garlic, and Parmesan cheese. For a little crunch, add some croutons.

## 6.2   Hearty Soups and Stews

Soups and stews are comforting and can be made in large batches for easy lunches throughout the week. Here are some hearty options:

### 1. Lentil Soup

Cook lentils with diced carrots, celery, onion, and garlic in a vegetable broth. Add tomatoes and spices like cumin and turmeric for flavor. This soup is high in fiber and protein, making it a perfect lunch option.

### 2. Chicken and Vegetable Stew

Simmer chicken breasts with carrots, potatoes, peas, and green beans in a chicken broth. Season with herbs like thyme and rosemary. This stew is hearty and filling, ideal for a satisfying lunch.

### 3. Butternut Squash Soup

Roast butternut squash cubes and blend them with vegetable broth, onion, garlic, and a touch of coconut milk. Season with nutmeg and cinnamon for a warm, comforting soup that's perfect for fall or winter.

### 4. Beef and Barley Stew

Cook beef chunks with barley, carrots, onions, and celery in a beef broth. Add bay leaves and thyme for extra flavor. This stew is rich and filling, making it a great option for a hearty lunch.

## 6.3 Delicious Sandwiches and Wraps

Sandwiches and wraps are versatile and can be packed with a variety of healthy ingredients. Here are some delicious recipes:

## 1. Turkey and Avocado Wrap

Spread a whole grain wrap with hummus and top with sliced turkey, avocado, lettuce, and tomato. Roll up and slice in half for a quick and easy lunch.

## 2. Mediterranean Veggie Sandwich

Layer hummus, roasted red peppers, cucumber slices, spinach, and feta cheese between two slices of whole grain bread. This sandwich is flavorful and packed with nutrients.

## 3. Chicken Salad Wrap

Mix shredded chicken with Greek yogurt, celery, grapes, and a touch of Dijon mustard. Spoon into a whole grain wrap and add lettuce for crunch. This wrap is high in protein and perfect for lunch on the go.

## 4. Tuna Salad Sandwich

Combine canned tuna with avocado, lemon juice, and diced red onion. Top with tomato and lettuce and spread over whole grain bread. This sandwich is a healthy twist on a classic favorite.

## 6.4 Vegetarian and Vegan Options

For those following a vegetarian or vegan diet, here are some delicious and nutritious lunch options:

### 1. Vegan Buddha Bowl

Combine cooked quinoa, roasted sweet potatoes, chickpeas, avocado, and sautéed kale in a bowl. Drizzle with tahini dressing and sprinkle with sesame seeds. This bowl is flavorful and nutrient-rich.

### 2. Chickpea Salad Sandwich

Mash chickpeas with avocado, lemon juice, and diced red onion. Top with tomato and lettuce and spread over whole grain bread. This sandwich is a great plant-based alternative to traditional chicken or tuna salad.

## 3. Veggie Stir-Fry

Sauté a variety of vegetables like bell peppers, broccoli, carrots, and snap peas in a bit of olive oil. Add tofu or tempeh for protein and toss with a soy sauce and ginger dressing. Serve with brown rice for a full dinner.

## 4. Lentil and Veggie Wrap

Cook lentils with diced carrots, celery, and onions. Spoon into a whole grain wrap and top with avocado and a drizzle of tahini dressing. This wrap is high in fiber and protein, making it a satisfying lunch option.

By incorporating these breakfast and lunch recipes into your daily routine, you can support your health and manage PCOS symptoms more effectively. The following chapters will provide even more delicious recipes and tips to help you on your journey to better health.

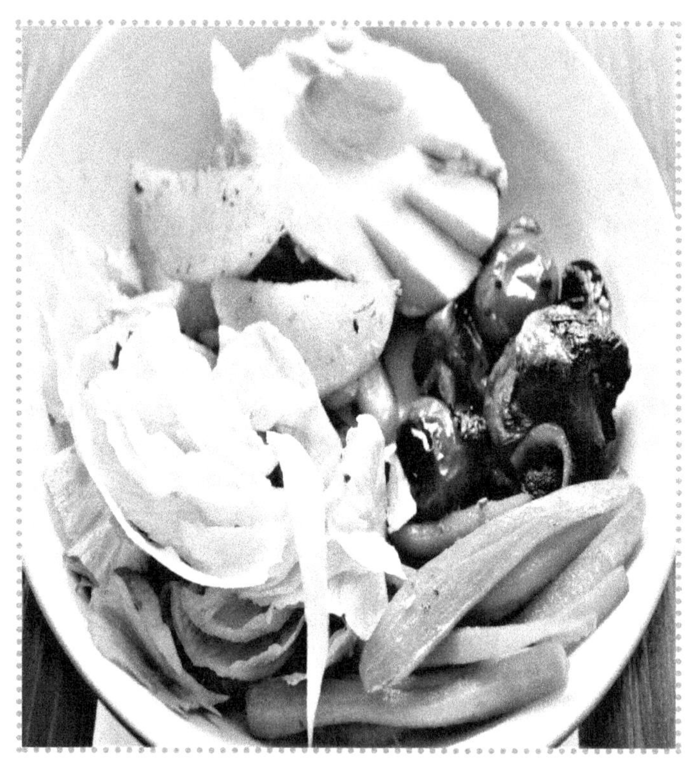

# CHAPTER SEVEN

## Dinner Recipes

Dinner is an essential meal that offers an opportunity to relax and refuel after a busy day. For those managing PCOS, a nutritious and well-balanced dinner can help stabilize blood sugar levels overnight and prepare the body for restful sleep. This chapter will provide a variety of dinner recipes focusing on balanced and flavorful main courses, lean proteins, nutritious sides and vegetables, and convenient slow cooker and one-pot meals.

## 7.1    Balanced and Flavorful Main Courses

Creating a balanced dinner means including a good mix of protein, healthy fats, and carbohydrates. Here are some recipes that are not only nutritious but also bursting with flavor.

## 1. Grilled Lemon Herb Chicken

Marinate chicken breasts in a mixture of olive oil, lemon juice, garlic, and herbs like rosemary and thyme. Grill until cooked through and serve with a side of quinoa and steamed broccoli. This dish is light, flavorful, and rich in lean protein.

## 2. Baked Salmon with Dill and Lemon

Place salmon filets on a baking sheet and season with olive oil, lemon juice, fresh dill, salt, and pepper. Bake at 375°F (190°C) for about 20 minutes or until the fish flakes easily with a fork. Serve with a side of roasted Brussels sprouts and a wild rice blend for a balanced meal.

## 3. Stuffed Bell Peppers

Remove the seeds from bell peppers by cutting off the tops. In a skillet, sauté onions, garlic, and lean ground turkey. Add cooked quinoa, black beans, corn, and diced tomatoes. Stuff the mixture into the bell peppers and bake at 350°F (175°C) for 30 minutes. If wanted, put some cheese on top. These peppers are a great source of protein, fiber, and vegetables.

## 4. Eggplant Parmesan

Slice eggplant and bake until tender. Layer the eggplant slices with marinara sauce and part-skim mozzarella cheese in a baking dish. Bake at 375°F (190°C) until the cheese is melted and bubbly. Serve with a side salad for a delicious and comforting vegetarian dinner.

## 7.2 Lean Proteins: Chicken, Fish, and Plant-Based Options

Incorporating lean proteins into your diet is crucial for managing PCOS symptoms. Here are some dinner recipes featuring chicken, fish, and plant-based proteins.

## 1. Chicken Stir-Fry

Sauté chicken breast strips with an assortment of vegetables like bell peppers, broccoli, and snap peas in a bit of olive oil. Add soy sauce, ginger, and garlic for flavor. Serve over brown rice or quinoa for a high-protein, low-fat dinner.

## 2. Baked Cod with Tomatoes and Olives

Place cod filets in a baking dish and top with diced tomatoes, olives, capers, and a drizzle of olive oil. Bake at 375°F (190°C) for 20-25 minutes or until the fish is opaque and flakes easily. Serve with a side of roasted sweet potatoes and green beans.

## 3. Lentil and Vegetable Stew

In a large pot, sauté onions, garlic, carrots, and celery in olive oil. Add lentils, diced tomatoes, vegetable broth, and spices like cumin and turmeric. Simmer until the lentils are tender. This stew is rich in plant-based protein and fiber, making it a hearty and satisfying dinner.

## 4. Tofu and Vegetable Curry

Sauté tofu cubes with onions, garlic, and ginger. Incorporate an assortment of veggies such as spinach, bell peppers, and zucchini. Stir in coconut milk and curry paste, and simmer until the vegetables are tender. Serve over brown rice for a flavorful and protein-rich dinner.

## 7.3   Sides and Vegetables

A nutritious dinner is incomplete without healthy sides and vegetables. Here are some recipes to complement your main courses.

## 1. Roasted Vegetables

Toss an assortment of vegetables like carrots, parsnips, and Brussels sprouts with olive oil, salt, and pepper. Roast at 400°F (200°C) for 25-30 minutes, stirring halfway through, until the vegetables are tender and caramelized.

## 2. Quinoa Pilaf

Cook quinoa according to package instructions. In a skillet, sauté diced onions, garlic, and bell peppers in olive oil. Stir in the cooked quinoa, and add a handful of chopped fresh herbs like parsley and dill. This is a high-fiber, high-protein side dish.

### 3. Garlic Mashed Cauliflower

Steam cauliflower florets until tender. Blend with a bit of olive oil, garlic, salt, and pepper until smooth. This mashed cauliflower is a low-carb alternative to mashed potatoes and pairs well with a variety of main courses.

### 4. Green Bean Almondine

Sauté green beans in olive oil with sliced almonds and a squeeze of lemon juice. This simple side dish is not only nutritious but also adds a delightful crunch to your dinner plate.

## 7.4 Slow Cooker and One-Pot Meals

Slow cooker and one-pot meals are perfect for busy individuals, allowing you to prepare nutritious dinners with minimal effort. These are a few quick and tasty dishes.

# 1. Slow Cooker Chicken and Vegetable Stew

Combine chicken thighs, diced potatoes, carrots, celery, onions, and garlic in a slow cooker. Add chicken broth, thyme, and bay leaves. Cook the chicken for 6 to 8 hours on low, or until it is tender. This stew is hearty, comforting, and requires minimal prep time.

# 1. One-Pot Pasta with Vegetables

In a large pot, combine whole grain pasta, diced tomatoes, spinach, garlic, and vegetable broth. Bring to a boil and simmer until the pasta is cooked and the liquid is mostly absorbed. Stir in a bit of Parmesan cheese before serving. This one-pot meal is easy to make and packed with nutrients.

# 2. Slow Cooker Lentil Soup

Combine lentils, diced carrots, celery, onions, garlic, and vegetable broth in a slow cooker. Add spices like cumin, coriander, and turmeric. Cook the lentils for 6 to 8 hours on low, or until they are soft. This soup is rich in plant-based protein and fiber, making it a perfect dinner option.

## 3. One-Pot Chicken and Rice

In a large pot, sauté chicken thighs with onions, garlic, and bell peppers. Add brown rice, chicken broth, and a can of diced tomatoes. Bring to a boil, then reduce heat and simmer until the rice is cooked and the liquid is absorbed. This one-pot meal is flavorful and satisfying.

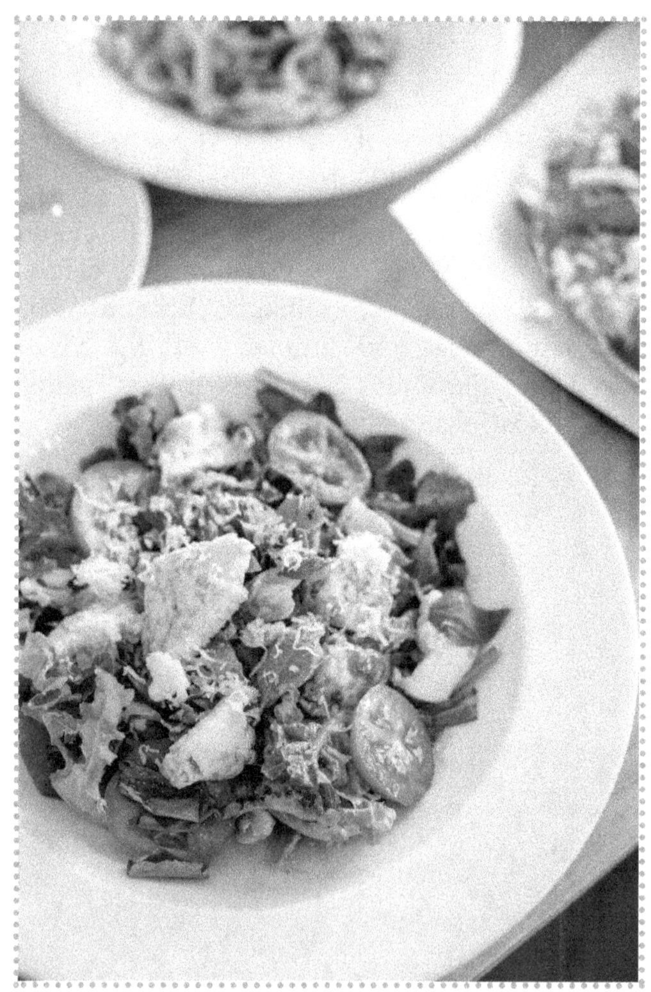

# CHAPTER EIGHT

## Snacks and Appetizers

Snacks and appetizers are important for keeping energy levels stable and preventing overeating during meals. This chapter offers a variety of healthy snacking ideas, finger foods for gatherings, dips and spreads, and on-the-go snack options.

## 8.1   Healthy Snacking Ideas

Healthy snacks can help manage hunger and provide essential nutrients between meals. Here are some nutritious snacking ideas:

### 1. Apple Slices with Almond Butter

Slice an apple and serve with a tablespoon of almond butter. This snack is quick, easy, and provides a good balance of protein, healthy fats, and fiber.

## 2. Greek Yogurt with Berries

Top a bowl of Greek yogurt with fresh berries and a drizzle of honey. This snack is high in protein and antioxidants, making it a perfect option for a mid-morning or afternoon pick-me-up.

## 3. Veggie Sticks with Hummus

Cut up a variety of vegetables like carrots, celery, and bell peppers. Serve with a side of hummus for a crunchy and satisfying snack that's rich in fiber and healthy fats.

## 4. Mixed Nuts and Seeds

Create a custom mix of nuts and seeds like almonds, walnuts, and pumpkin seeds. Portion into small bags for a convenient, nutrient-dense snack that's easy to take on the go.

## 8.2  Finger Foods for Gatherings

When hosting gatherings, it's important to offer snacks that are both delicious and nutritious. Here are some finger food ideas that are perfect for entertaining:

### 1. Caprese Skewers

Cherry tomatoes, mozzarella balls, and fresh basil leaves should all be threaded onto skewers. Drizzle with balsamic glaze before serving. These skewers are easy to make and always a hit at parties.

### 2. Cucumber and Smoked Salmon Bites

Slice cucumbers into rounds and top with a bit of cream cheese and a piece of smoked salmon. Garnish with fresh dill. These bites are elegant, light, and full of flavor.

## 3. Mini Stuffed Bell Peppers

Remove the seeds after halving the small bell peppers. Fill with a mixture of quinoa, black beans, corn, and diced tomatoes. These mini peppers are colorful, nutritious, and perfect for snacking.

## 4. Sweet Potato Rounds with Avocado

Slice sweet potatoes into rounds and roast until tender. Top with mashed avocado and a sprinkle of chili flakes. These rounds are a delicious and healthy alternative to traditional chips and dip.

## 8.3 Dips and Spreads

Dips and spreads can elevate any snack or appetizer. Here are some healthy options that are easy to prepare and packed with flavor:

## 1. Classic Hummus

Add the chickpeas, tahini, olive oil, lemon juice, and garlic and blend until smooth. Accompany with whole grain crackers or fresh vegetables. Hummus is a versatile dip that's rich in protein and healthy fats.

## 2. Guacamole

Mash ripe avocados with lime juice, diced red onion, chopped cilantro, and a pinch of salt. Serve with tortilla chips or vegetable sticks. Guacamole is creamy, flavorful, and loaded with healthy fats.

## 3. Spinach and Artichoke Dip

Sauté spinach and artichoke hearts with garlic in a bit of olive oil. Blend with Greek yogurt, Parmesan cheese, and a touch of lemon juice. This dip is creamy and delicious, perfect for spreading on whole grain toast or dipping with vegetables.

## 4. Roasted Red Pepper Dip

Blend roasted red peppers with Greek yogurt, garlic, and a bit of olive oil until smooth. This dip is smoky, tangy, and pairs well with pita bread or veggie sticks.

## 8.4   On-the-Go Snack Options

### 1. For those busy days

When you're constantly on the move, having healthy snacks on hand is essential. Here are some convenient on-the-go snack options:

### 1. Trail Mix

Create a custom trail mix with your favorite nuts, seeds, dried fruits, and a bit of dark chocolate. Portion into small bags for an easy and portable snack that's full of energy-boosting nutrients.

## 2. Energy Balls

Mix oats, nut butter, honey, and add-ins like chia seeds, flaxseeds, and dried fruit. Roll into bite-sized balls and refrigerate. These energy balls are ideal as a light snack or an energy boost before working out.

## 3. Protein Bars

Choose or make protein bars with minimal added sugars and natural ingredients. Look for bars that contain a good balance of protein, healthy fats, and fiber to keep you full and energized.

## 4. Fresh Fruit

Keep fresh fruit like apples, bananas, or oranges on hand for a quick and easy snack. Fresh fruit is naturally sweet, hydrating, and provides essential vitamins and minerals.

By incorporating these dinner, snack, and appetizer recipes into your routine, you can support your health and manage PCOS symptoms more effectively. The following chapters will provide even more delicious recipes and tips to help you on your journey to better health.

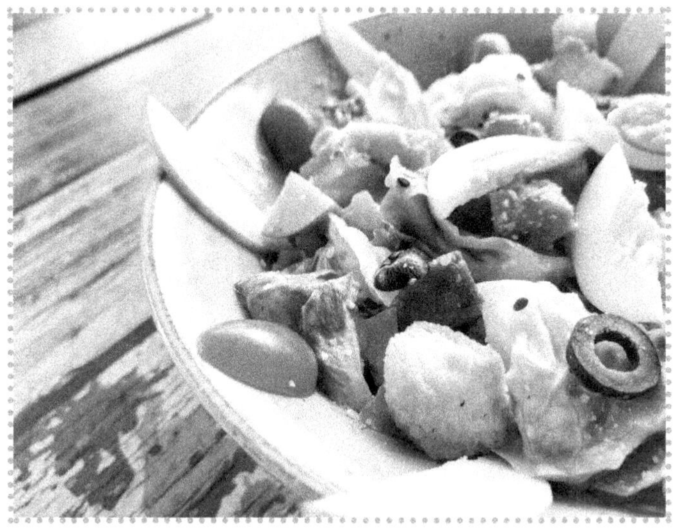

# CHAPTER NINE

## Desserts

Desserts can be a delightful way to end a meal, but they often come laden with sugar and unhealthy fats. For those managing PCOS, it's crucial to enjoy sweet treats that support rather than hinder your health goals. In this chapter, we'll explore desserts that offer a healthy twist, focus on fruit-based options, and provide low-sugar, low-carb, and guilt-free indulgences. These recipes will allow you to satisfy your sweet tooth while staying on track with your health.

## 9.1 Sweet Treats with a Healthy Twist

### 1. Avocado Chocolate Mousse

Avocado might seem like an unusual ingredient for a dessert, but it provides a creamy texture and healthy fats. Blend ripe avocados with unsweetened cocoa powder, a bit of honey or maple syrup, and a splash of vanilla extract. Refrigerate for a few hours before serving. This mousse is rich, chocolaty, and much healthier than traditional versions.

## 2. Greek Yogurt Parfait

Layer Greek yogurt with fresh berries, a drizzle of honey, and a sprinkle of granola or nuts. This parfait is not only visually appealing but also rich in protein and antioxidants. It makes for a quick and easy dessert that can also double as a nutritious breakfast.

## 3. Chia Seed Pudding

Mix chia seeds with unsweetened almond milk and a touch of vanilla extract. Let it sit overnight in the refrigerator until it reaches a pudding-like consistency. Top with fresh fruits, nuts, or a bit of dark chocolate for added flavor. Chia seeds are packed with omega-3 fatty acids, fiber, and protein, making this dessert a nutritional powerhouse.

## 4. Banana Nice Cream

Freeze ripe bananas and blend them until smooth. You can add a splash of almond milk to help with blending. For extra flavor, mix in cocoa powder, vanilla extract, or a handful of berries. This banana "nice cream" is a delicious, dairy-free, and guilt-free alternative to traditional ice cream.

## 9.2   Fruit-Based Desserts

## 1. Baked Apples with Cinnamon

Core apples and place them in a baking dish. Fill the centers with a mixture of oats, nuts, and a bit of honey. Sprinkle with cinnamon and bake at 350°F (175°C) until tender. These baked apples are warm, comforting, and perfect for a cozy dessert.

## 2. Berry Compote

Cook a mixture of fresh or frozen berries in a saucepan with a splash of water and a bit of honey or maple syrup. Simmer until the berries soften and develop into a viscous sauce. Serve warm over Greek yogurt, oatmeal, or on its own. Berry compote is a versatile and antioxidant-rich dessert option.

## 3. Grilled Peaches

Cut peaches in half and remove the pits. Grill them until tender and slightly caramelized. Drizzle some honey and a dollop of Greek yogurt on top. Grilled peaches are a simple yet elegant dessert that highlights the natural sweetness of the fruit.

## 4. Tropical Fruit Salad

Combine diced mango, pineapple, kiwi, and papaya in a bowl. Squeeze fresh lime juice over the fruit and add a sprinkle of shredded coconut. This tropical fruit salad is refreshing, vibrant, and full of vitamins and minerals.

## 9.3 Low-Sugar and Low-Carb Options

### 1. Almond Flour Cookies

Mix almond flour, a bit of coconut oil, an egg, and a sweetener like stevia or erythritol. Add a touch of vanilla extract and a handful of dark chocolate chips. Bake at 350°F (175°C) until golden brown. These cookies are low in carbs and sugar, making them a great option for satisfying a sweet craving without spiking your blood sugar.

### 2. Coconut Macaroons

Blend shredded coconut with egg whites and a bit of honey. Form into small mounds and bake at

325°F (160°C) until golden. These macaroons are chewy, sweet, and low in sugar, perfect for a light dessert or snack.

## 3. Dark Chocolate Bark

Melt dark chocolate and spread it thinly on a parchment-lined baking sheet. Sprinkle with nuts, seeds, and dried fruits. Let it set in the refrigerator until firm, then break into pieces. This chocolate bark is a delicious way to enjoy a treat that's rich in antioxidants and healthy fats.

## 4. Sugar-Free Jello

Make homemade jello using gelatin and a natural sweetener like stevia. Add fresh fruit pieces before chilling. This jello is a fun, low-calorie dessert that's easy to make and customize with your favorite flavors.

## 9.4  Guilt-Free Indulgences

### 1.  Oatmeal Raisin Energy Bites

Combine rolled oats, almond butter, honey, and raisins. Shape into bite-sized spheres and chill until solid. These energy bites are a perfect on-the-go treat that provides a good balance of carbohydrates, protein, and healthy fats.

### 2.  Pumpkin Spice Muffins

Mix canned pumpkin, almond flour, eggs, and a bit of maple syrup with pumpkin pie spice. Bake in muffin tins at 350°F (175°C) until a toothpick comes out clean. These muffins are moist, flavorful, and a great way to enjoy a seasonal treat without the guilt.

### 3.  Chocolate-Covered Strawberries

Dip fresh strawberries in melted dark chocolate and let them set on a parchment-lined tray. Refrigerate until the chocolate is firm. These chocolate-covered strawberries are elegant, delicious, and provide a perfect balance of sweetness and health benefits.


Lemon Coconut Bars

Mix almond flour, shredded coconut, and a bit of honey to form the crust. Blend lemon juice, zest, eggs, and a sweetener for the filling. Bake until set and refrigerate before cutting into bars. These lemon coconut bars are tangy, sweet, and satisfying, offering a refreshing dessert option.

# CHAPTER TEN

## Tips for Long-Term Success

Managing PCOS is a lifelong journey that involves maintaining healthy habits, staying motivated, and finding the right balance in your lifestyle. This chapter will provide valuable tips to help you stay on track, manage cravings and emotional eating, incorporate exercise and lifestyle changes, and access support and resources for PCOS management.

## 10.1 Staying Motivated and On Track

### 1. Set Realistic Goals

Setting achievable goals is crucial for long-term success. Start with small, manageable changes and gradually build on them. For example, aim to incorporate one new healthy recipe each week or add an extra 10 minutes to your daily walk. Celebrating these small victories can boost your motivation and confidence.

## 2. Keep a Food Journal

Tracking what you eat can help you stay mindful of your choices and identify patterns. Use a food journal to record your meals, snacks, and any symptoms you experience. This can help you understand which foods support your health and which may trigger symptoms.

## 3. Find Your Why

Understanding your motivation for managing PCOS is essential. Whether it's improving your energy levels, managing weight, or enhancing your fertility, keeping your reasons in mind can help you stay focused and committed to your goals.

## 4. Reward Yourself

Celebrate your progress with non-food rewards. Treat yourself to a relaxing spa day, a new workout outfit, or a fun activity you enjoy. Rewards can help reinforce positive behaviors and keep you motivated.

## 10.2     Managing Cravings and Emotional Eating

### 1. Identify Triggers

Recognize what triggers your cravings or emotional eating. Stress, boredom, and certain social situations can all play a role. Once you identify your triggers, you can develop strategies to manage them, such as practicing stress-relief techniques or finding alternative activities to distract yourself.

### 2. Plan Ahead

Prepare healthy snacks and meals in advance to reduce the temptation to reach for unhealthy options. Keep nutritious snacks like nuts, fresh fruit, and yogurt on hand so you have something healthy to turn to when cravings strike.

## 3. Practice Mindful Eating

Eating mindfully is taking time to appreciate each bite, eating slowly, and paying attention to your body's signals of hunger and fullness. You can lessen emotional eating and have a better relationship with food by engaging in this exercise.

## 4. Seek Support

Talking to a therapist or joining a support group can provide valuable tools and encouragement for managing emotional eating. Sharing your experiences with others who understand can help you feel less alone and more empowered to make positive changes.

## 10.3    Exercise and Lifestyle Changes

### 1. Find Activities You Enjoy

Incorporating physical activity into your routine is crucial for managing PCOS, but it's important to choose activities you enjoy. Whether it's dancing, swimming, hiking, or yoga, finding exercise that you look forward to can make it easier to stick with it.

### 2. Create a Balanced Routine

Aim to include a mix of cardiovascular exercise, strength training, and flexibility exercises in your routine. Cardio activities like walking, running, or cycling can improve heart health, while strength training helps build muscle and boost metabolism. Flexibility exercises like stretching or yoga can enhance overall well-being.

### 3. Prioritize Sleep

Quality sleep is essential for managing PCOS and overall health. Make sure your bedroom is restful, stick to a regular sleep schedule, and have a calming nighttime ritual. Try to get seven to nine hours each night.

### 4. Manage Stress

Chronic stress can exacerbate PCOS symptoms, so it's important to find effective ways to manage it. Practice stress-relief techniques such as deep breathing, meditation, or spending time in nature. Regular physical activity and adequate sleep also play a significant role in stress management.

## 10.4 Support and Resources for PCOS Management

### 1. Join a Support Group

Connecting with others who are managing PCOS can provide emotional support and practical advice. Look for local or online support groups where you can share experiences, learn from others, and find encouragement.

### 2. Consult a Healthcare Professional

Working with a healthcare professional who understands PCOS can provide valuable guidance. A registered dietitian, endocrinologist, or gynecologist can help you develop a personalized plan for managing your symptoms and improving your overall health.

## 3. Use Technology

Numerous apps and internet tools are available to assist you in keeping track of your progress, find healthy recipes, and stay motivated. Explore tools that can help you manage your diet, exercise routine, and overall well-being.

## 4. Educate Yourself

Continuing to learn about PCOS and how it affects your body can empower you to make informed decisions about your health. Read books, attend workshops, and stay up-to-date with the latest research and recommendations.

By implementing these tips and strategies, you can create a sustainable and healthy lifestyle that supports your long-term success in managing PCOS. Remember that every small step you take brings you closer to better health and well-being. The following chapters will provide even more insights and practical advice to help you on your journey.

# CONCLUSION

I'm grateful that you're traveling with me through the "PCOS Diet Cookbook for Beginners". You know a ton by now about controlling PCOS with a healthy, well-balanced diet. With knowledge of the fundamentals of PCOS and delectable recipes for every meal, you are prepared to take charge of your health and wellbeing.

Recall that living with PCOS means having to be patient, persistent, and having an optimistic outlook on life. To support your health objectives, develop a sustainable lifestyle using the strategies, recipes, and advice in this book.

Remain inspired, continue attempting new dishes, and—above all—pay attention to your body. By using proactive measures and appropriate resources, you can successfully manage your PCOS and lead a happy, healthy life.

I appreciate you include me on your trip. Cheers to your well-being and prosperity!

www.ingramcontent.com/pod-product-compliance
Lightning Source LLC
Chambersburg PA
CBHW051648250726
48653CB00007B/2551